# COOKING FOR PROSTATE HEALTH

## Conquering Prostate Cancer Naturally, Without Requiring Any Surgical Procedure

*100+ Tasty and Effortless Recipes for Prostate Wellness*

By

**Jerome Woodworth**

# TABLE OF CONTENTS

## Introduction

Anderson had always been a health-conscious individual, but when he received a diagnosis of prostate problems, he realized he needed to take his health to the next level. He started researching ways to improve prostate health and discovered a book titled "100+ Tasty and Effortless Recipes for Prostate Wellness: Cooking for Prostate Health."

Excited about the prospect of improving his health through diet, Anderson eagerly dove into the book and began incorporating the delicious and healthy recipes into his daily routine. He was amazed at how easy the recipes were to prepare and how tasty they were. He quickly found that he didn't have to sacrifice flavour for health, and he started enjoying meals more than ever before.

As he continued to follow the recipes in the book, Anderson noticed significant improvements in his prostate health. His symptoms began to subside, and his energy levels increased. He felt healthier and happier than he had in years, and he knew that the recipes in the book were the reason why.

Anderson continued to follow the book's recipes and recommendations for several months, and he was ecstatic when he went in for his follow-up appointment with his doctor. His prostate problems had completely cleared up, and his doctor was impressed with his progress. Anderson couldn't believe that something as simple as changing his diet could have such a significant impact on his health.

Today, Anderson continues to use the book's recipes to maintain his prostate health, and he recommends the book to anyone who is looking to improve their health through diet. He knows first-hand the power of healthy and delicious food and is grateful for the positive impact that

"100+ Tasty and Effortless Recipes for Prostate Wellness: Cooking for Prostate Health" had on his life.

Prostate health is an issue that affects many men as they age. According to the American Cancer Society, one in eight men will be diagnosed with prostate cancer at some point in their lives. While there is no guaranteed way to prevent prostate problems, research has shown that a healthy diet can help reduce the risk of prostate cancer and improve overall prostate health.

*"100+ Tasty and Effortless Recipes for Prostate Wellness"*: Cooking for Prostate Health" is a comprehensive cookbook that provides delicious and nutritious recipes to support prostate health. This book is designed to help men take charge of their health by incorporating easy-to-prepare and flavourful recipes into their diet.

The recipes in this book are carefully crafted to include ingredients that are known to support prostate health, such **as tomatoes, broccoli, salmon**, **and nuts.** The book also provides a detailed explanation of the nutrients that are essential for prostate health and tips on how to prepare food in a way that maximizes its nutritional benefits.

In addition to providing tasty and nutritious recipes, "100+ Tasty and Effortless Recipes for Prostate Wellness: Cooking for Prostate Health" also educates readers on the basics of prostate health. The book explains what the prostate is, common prostate problems, and how diet can affect prostate health. It also provides guidance on foods to avoid and cooking methods to use to ensure optimal prostate health.

This cookbook is perfect for anyone looking to improve their prostate health through diet, whether they are currently experiencing prostate problems or want to take proactive measures to reduce their risk. The recipes are easy to follow, delicious, and packed with nutrients that are essential for prostate health.

Overall, "100+ Tasty and Effortless Recipes for Prostate Wellness: Cooking for Prostate Health" is an essential resource for men who want to

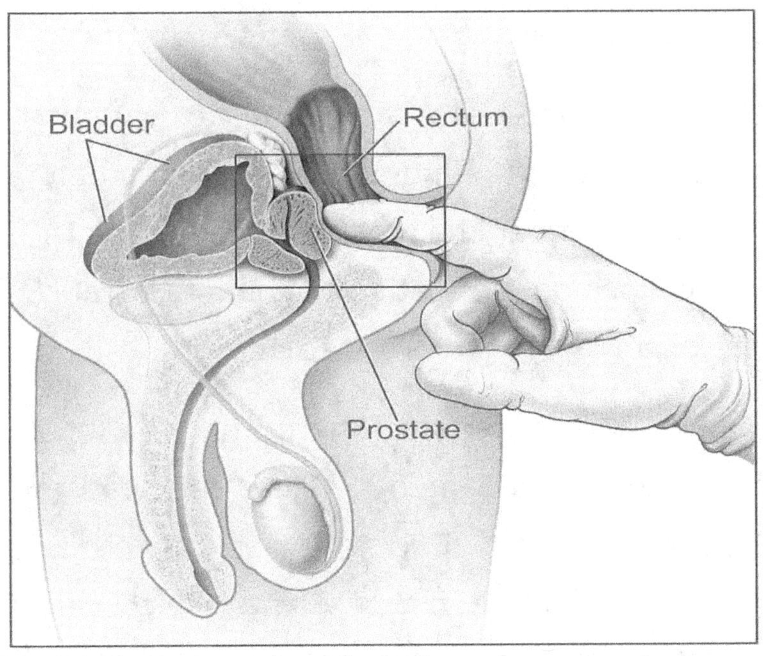



take control of their health and improve their prostate health through tasty and effortless recipes.

# CHAPTER 1

## Understanding Prostate Health

Prostate health is a crucial aspect of men's health, and it is essential to understand what it is and how it can affect our lives. The prostate is a gland that is part of the male reproductive system, and it plays an important role in producing and transporting semen.

Prostate problems can arise due to various reasons, including inflammation, enlargement, and cancer. Some of the most common prostate problems include prostatitis, benign prostatic hyperplasia (BPH), and prostate cancer.

Prostatitis is a condition where the prostate gland becomes inflamed, which can cause discomfort and pain. BPH is a non-cancerous enlargement of the prostate gland, which can cause difficulty in urination, urinary frequency, and other related symptoms. Prostate cancer, on the other hand, is a potentially life-threatening condition that occurs when the cells in the prostate gland grow uncontrollably.

It is essential to understand the symptoms and risk factors associated with prostate problems to identify them early and seek timely medical attention. Some of the symptoms of prostate problems include difficulty urinating, frequent urination, pain or discomfort during urination, blood in the urine or semen, and pain or discomfort in the lower back or pelvic area.

Several factors can increase the risk of developing prostate problems, including age, family history, and diet. Research has shown that certain dietary habits, such as consuming high amounts of red meat, saturated fats, and processed foods, can increase the risk of prostate problems.

On the other hand, a diet rich in fruits, vegetables, whole grains, and healthy fats, such as those found in fish, nuts, and seeds, can help improve prostate health and reduce the risk of prostate problems.

It is crucial to take proactive measures to maintain optimal prostate health by adopting healthy lifestyle habits such as regular exercise, a balanced diet, and regular check-ups with a healthcare professional.

In conclusion, understanding prostate health is crucial for men of all ages. By educating ourselves about the prostate, its functions, and potential problems, we can take proactive steps to maintain good prostate health and prevent the onset of prostate problems. Regular check-ups with healthcare professionals and adopting healthy lifestyle habits can help reduce the risk of developing prostate problems and ensure a healthy and happy life.

## What is the prostate?

An organ called the prostate is a component of the male reproductive system. It is a small, walnut-sized gland that is located just below the bladder and in front of the rectum. The prostate gland surrounds the urethra, which is the tube that carries urine and semen out of the body.

The primary function of the prostate gland is to produce and secrete a fluid that makes up a significant portion of semen. The fluid helps to nourish and transport sperm during ejaculation, which is necessary for fertilization.

The prostate gland is a complex organ made up of several types of cells, including glandular cells that produce the fluid, muscle cells that help to contract and expel the fluid during ejaculation, and stromal cells that provide support and structure to the gland.

Prostate problems can occur when the cells in the gland grow uncontrollably, leading to an enlarged prostate or prostate cancer. Benign prostatic hyperplasia (BPH), a non-cancerous enlargement of the prostate gland, is a common condition that affects many men as they age.

Prostate cancer is a potentially life-threatening condition that occurs when the cells in the prostate gland grow uncontrollably and form a tumor. One of the most typical cancers in males is prostate cancer, and effective treatment depends on early detection.

Regular check-ups with healthcare professionals can help to detect prostate problems early on and prevent the onset of serious conditions. Men should be aware of the potential symptoms of prostate problems, such as difficulty urinating, frequent urination, pain or discomfort during urination, blood in the urine or semen, and pain or discomfort in the lower back or pelvic area.

In conclusion, the prostate gland is an essential part of the male reproductive system that plays a crucial role in the production and transport of semen. Understanding the anatomy and function of the prostate gland is crucial for maintaining good prostate health and preventing the onset of prostate problems. Regular check-ups with healthcare professionals can help detect prostate problems early on and ensure timely treatment.

## Common prostate problems:

The prostate gland is a small, walnut-shaped gland located in the male reproductive system. It is responsible for producing seminal fluid, which helps to nourish and protect sperm. As men age, the prostate gland can undergo changes that can lead to various prostate problems. In this note, we will discuss some of the most common prostate problems, their symptoms, causes, and treatment options.

**Benign Prostatic Hyperplasia (BPH):**

BPH is a non-cancerous enlargement of the prostate gland. It is a common condition that affects men as they age, with up to 90% of men over the age of 80 having some degree of BPH. The enlarged prostate gland can put pressure on the urethra, leading to a range of symptoms such as:

- Difficulty starting or stopping urination
- Weak urine flow
- Need to urinate frequently, especially at night
- Incomplete emptying of the bladder
- Dribbling after urination

The exact cause of BPH is not fully understood, but it is believed to be related to hormonal changes that occur as men age. Treatment options for BPH include medications, minimally invasive procedures, or surgery.

**Prostatitis:**

Prostatitis is an inflammation of the prostate gland. It can be caused by a bacterial infection, a non-bacterial infection, or another underlying medical condition. Symptoms of prostatitis can vary but may include:

- Pain or discomfort in the groin or lower back
- Painful urination
- Urinary frequency and urgency
- Fever and chills
- Blood in the urine

Treatment for prostatitis depends on the underlying cause but may include antibiotics, pain relief medication, and lifestyle changes such as increasing fluid intake and avoiding spicy or acidic foods.

**Prostate Cancer:**

Prostate cancer is a type of cancer that occurs when abnormal cells grow and multiply in the prostate gland. Prostate cancer is one of the most common cancers in men, and the risk of developing it increases with age. Symptoms of prostate cancer can include:

- Difficulty urinating
- Blood in the urine or semen
- Pain or discomfort in the pelvic area
- Bone pain, especially in the hips, spine, or ribs

Treatment options for prostate cancer include surgery, radiation therapy, chemotherapy, and hormone therapy.

**Prostate Infection:**

A prostate infection can occur when bacteria or other microbes enter the prostate gland. Symptoms of a prostate infection can include:

- Painful urination
- Fever and chills
- Muscle aches
- Lower back or pelvic pain
- Urinary frequency and urgency

*Antibiotics are typically used to treat a prostate infection.*

**Prostate Stones:**

Prostate stones are small, hard mineral deposits that can form in the prostate gland. They are typically not harmful but can cause pain, discomfort, and difficulty urinating. Treatment for prostate stones may include medication to relieve pain, antibiotics to treat infection, or minimally invasive procedures to remove the stones.

In conclusion, prostate problems are common among men, especially as they age. Regular prostate check-ups and screening can help to detect and treat prostate problems early, improving outcomes and quality of life. Men should speak with their healthcare provider if they experience any symptoms or concerns related to their prostate health.

**How diet affects prostate health:**

The prostate gland is a small, walnut-shaped gland located in the male reproductive system. It is responsible for producing seminal fluid, which helps to nourish and protect sperm. As men age, the prostate gland can undergo changes that can lead to various prostate problems. In this note, we will discuss some of the most common prostate problems, their symptoms, causes, and treatment options.

**Fruits and Vegetables:**

A diet rich in fruits and vegetables is essential for prostate health. These foods contain antioxidants and other nutrients that can help to prevent cellular damage and reduce inflammation in the body. The phytochemicals found in fruits and vegetables have been linked to a reduced risk of prostate cancer. Examples of fruits and vegetables that are good for prostate health include:

- Tomatoes
- Broccoli
- Cauliflower
- Kale
- Berries
- Citrus fruits
- Apples
- Pomegranates

**Healthy Fats:**

Omega-3 fatty acids, which are found in fatty fish such as salmon, tuna, and sardines, have been shown to reduce inflammation and may lower the risk of developing prostate cancer. Nuts, seeds, and avocados are also good sources of healthy fats and can be included in a prostate-healthy diet.

**Whole Grains:**

Whole grains are an excellent source of fiber, which can help to regulate bowel movements and reduce the risk of constipation. A diet rich in whole grains has been linked to a reduced risk of developing prostate cancer. Examples of whole grains include:

- Brown rice
- Quinoa
- Oatmeal
- Barley
- Whole wheat bread

- Whole grain pasta

**Red Meat and Dairy:**

High consumption of red meat and dairy products has been linked to an increased risk of prostate cancer. While it is not necessary to eliminate these foods completely, it is recommended to limit consumption and choose leaner cuts of meat and low-fat dairy products.

**Processed Foods and Sugars:**

A diet high in processed foods and sugars can lead to inflammation in the body, which has been linked to an increased risk of prostate cancer. It is recommended to limit the consumption of processed foods, sugary drinks, and sweets.

In conclusion, a healthy diet is essential for prostate health. Including a variety of fruits, vegetables, healthy fats, and whole grains in your diet while limiting red meat, dairy, processed foods, and sugars can help to promote prostate health and reduce the risk of developing prostate problems. For individualized dietary advice, speak with a medical professional or certified dietitian.

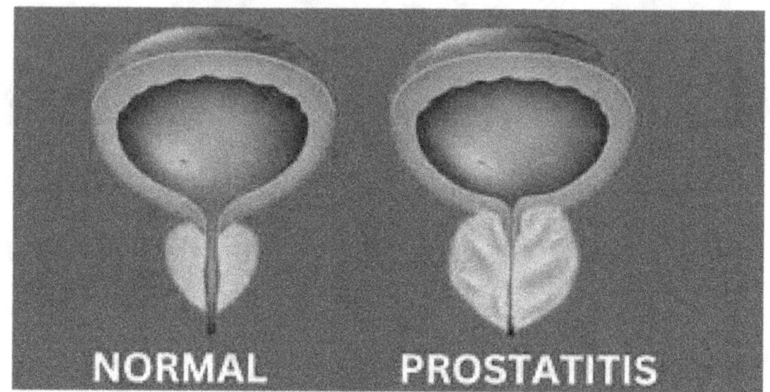


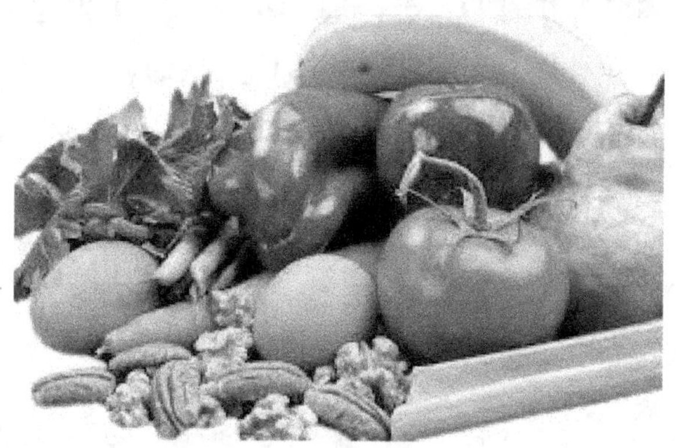

Diet for prostate cancer prevention

## CHAPTER 2:

**The Basics of Prostate-Healthy Eating:**

The prostate is a small gland located in the male reproductive system that plays an important role in reproductive health. Men are more likely to develop prostate issues as they mature. A healthy diet can help to support prostate health and reduce the risk of developing prostate problems. In this note, we will discuss the basics of prostate-healthy eating and provide tips for incorporating prostate-healthy foods into your diet.

**Include Fruits and Vegetables:**

Fruits and vegetables are an essential part of a prostate-healthy diet. These foods are rich in vitamins, minerals, and antioxidants that can help to reduce inflammation and prevent cellular damage. Make an effort to eat a range of fruits and vegetables, such as:

- Tomatoes
- Broccoli
- Cauliflower
- Kale
- Berries
- Citrus fruits
- Apples
- Pomegranates

**Choose Healthy Fats:**

Healthy fats, such as omega-3 fatty acids, can help to reduce inflammation in the body and promote prostate health. Include fatty fish like salmon, sardines, and tuna, nuts and seeds like walnuts and chia seeds, and healthy oils like olive oil in your diet.

**Consume Whole Grains:**

Whole grains are an excellent source of fibre, which can help to regulate bowel movements and reduce the risk of constipation. A diet rich in whole grains has been linked to a reduced risk of developing prostate cancer. Examples of whole grains include:

- Brown rice
- Quinoa
- Oatmeal
- Barley
- Whole wheat bread
- Whole grain pasta

**Limit Red Meat and Dairy:**

High consumption of red meat and dairy products has been linked to an increased risk of prostate cancer. While it is not necessary to eliminate these foods completely, it is recommended to limit consumption and choose leaner cuts of meat and low-fat dairy products.

**Reduce Processed Foods and Sugars:**

A diet high in processed foods and sugars can lead to inflammation in the body, which has been linked to an increased risk of prostate cancer. It is recommended to limit the consumption of processed foods, sugary drinks, and sweets.

**Stay Hydrated:**

Drinking enough water is essential for prostate health. Aim to drink at least 8-10 glasses of water per day to stay hydrated and support prostate health.

**Watch Your Portion Sizes:**

Eating too much food can lead to weight gain, which can increase the risk of developing prostate problems. Pay attention to your portion sizes and try to eat slowly to allow your body to feel full.

In conclusion, a prostate-healthy diet includes a variety of fruits, vegetables, healthy fats, whole grains, and limited amounts of red meat, dairy, processed foods, and sugars. Staying hydrated and watching portion sizes is also important for prostate health. For individualized dietary advice, speak with a medical professional or certified dietitian.

**Nutrients for prostate health:**

The prostate is a gland situated within the male reproductive system that generates a fluid responsible for the nourishment and safeguarding of sperm. It is crucial to sustain a healthy prostate for a man's general health and welfare.

Certain nutrients can play a crucial role in supporting prostate health. In this note, we will discuss the nutrients that are essential for prostate health and the foods that contain them.

## Zinc:

A vital mineral called zinc is important for the health of the prostate. It is involved in the production of testosterone and the growth and development of the prostate gland. Zinc is also important for immune system function and wound healing. Good food sources of zinc include:

- Oysters
- Beef
- Chicken
- Pork
- Yogurt
- Cheese
- Nuts

**Vitamin D**:

Vitamin D is required for bone health as well as immune system performance. It might also help to lower the chance of prostate cancer. The body can produce vitamin D when the skin is exposed to sunlight, but it can also be obtained from food sources such as:

- Fatty fish (salmon, tuna)

- Fortified dairy products
- Fortified cereals
- Vitamin E:

**Vitamin E** is an antioxidant that can help to prevent cellular damage and reduce inflammation in the body. It might also help to lower the chance of prostate cancer. Good food sources of vitamin E include:

- Almonds
- Sunflower seeds
- Avocado
- Spinach
- Sweet potatoes
- Wheat germ oil

**Selenium**:

Selenium is a mineral that is important for immune system function and may play a role in reducing the risk of prostate cancer. Good food sources of selenium include:

- Brazil nuts

- Tuna
- Chicken
- Brown rice
- Lentils

## Lycopene:

Lycopene is a powerful antioxidant that may play a role in reducing the risk of prostate cancer. It is found in high concentrations in tomatoes and tomato-based products such as:

- Tomato sauce
- Tomato juice
- Tomato paste

## Omega-3 Fatty Acids:

Omega-3 fatty acids are important for reducing inflammation in the body and may also play a role in reducing the risk of prostate cancer. Omega-3 fatty acid-rich foodstuffs include:

- Fatty fish (salmon, sardines, tuna)
- Flaxseed

- Chia seeds
- Walnuts

In conclusion, maintaining good prostate health is essential for overall male health and well-being. Consuming a diet rich in nutrients such as zinc, vitamin D, vitamin E, selenium, lycopene, and omega-3 fatty acids can help to support prostate health and reduce the risk of prostate problems. For individualized dietary advice, speak with a medical professional or certified dietitian.

**Foods to avoid:**

Prostate cancer is one of the most common types of cancer in men, and its risk increases with age. While there is no guaranteed way to prevent prostate cancer, a healthy diet can help reduce the risk and promote overall prostate health. On the other hand, certain foods have been linked to an increased risk of prostate cancer, and avoiding them can help reduce the risk. In this note, we will discuss foods to avoid to beat prostate cancer.

**Processed meats:**

Processed meats like hot dogs, sausages, and bacon contain high levels of saturated fat and preservatives, which have been linked to an increased risk of prostate cancer. It is recommended to limit the consumption of processed meats and opt for lean protein sources like chicken, fish, and plant-based protein alternatives like legumes.

**Dairy products:**

Dairy products, especially high-fat dairy products like whole milk, cheese, and butter, have been linked to an increased risk of prostate cancer. Studies have found that men who consume high amounts of dairy products have a higher risk of developing prostate cancer than those who consume low amounts. Instead of high-fat dairy products, try consuming low-fat or non-fat dairy products, like skim milk or yogurt.

**Red and processed meats:**

Red meat and processed meats have been linked to an increased risk of prostate cancer. Consuming high amounts of red meat or processed meats like beef, pork, lamb, or sausage can increase the risk of developing prostate cancer Choose lean protein sources instead, such as fish or poultry.

**Fried foods:**

Fried foods like French fries, fried chicken, and fried fish are high in fat and have been linked to an increased risk of prostate cancer. Fried foods are often cooked at high temperatures, which can create harmful compounds that may increase cancer risk. Instead, choose foods that are baked, roasted, or grilled.

**Sugary foods and drinks:**

High intake of sugary foods and drinks has been linked to an increased risk of prostate cancer. Consuming high amounts of sugar can lead to obesity, which is a risk factor for prostate cancer. Instead, choose foods that are low in sugar, such as fruits, vegetables, and whole grains.

In conclusion, maintaining a healthy diet that is low in processed meats, dairy products, red and processed meats, fried foods, and sugary foods and drinks can help reduce the risk of prostate cancer. Incorporating a variety of fruits, vegetables, whole grains, and lean protein sources can promote overall prostate health and help lower the risk of developing prostate cancer.

## Cooking methods for prostate health

Cooking methods can have a significant impact on the nutritional value of food, and choosing the right cooking methods can be beneficial for prostate health. Here are some cooking methods that can help promote prostate health:

## Grilling:

Grilling is a popular cooking method that can be beneficial for prostate health when done right. Grilling meat can help reduce the amount of fat in the meat, making it a healthier protein source. However, it is important to avoid overcooking the meat as this can create harmful compounds that may increase cancer risk. To minimize the formation of harmful compounds, it is recommended to marinate meat before grilling and avoid charring the meat.

**Steaming:**

Steaming is a healthy cooking method that can help retain the nutritional value of vegetables. Vegetables like broccoli, cauliflower, and kale are high in nutrients like vitamins A, C, and K, which are beneficial for prostate health. Steaming vegetables helps preserve their nutrients, making them an excellent addition to a prostate-healthy diet.

**Stir-frying:**

Stir-frying is a quick and healthy cooking method that can help retain the nutritional value of vegetables. When stir-frying vegetables, it is important to use a small amount of healthy oil like olive oil or coconut oil to prevent the vegetables from sticking to the pan. Adding spices and herbs like garlic, ginger, and turmeric can also help enhance the flavor of the dish and provide additional health benefits.

**Baking:**

Baking is a healthy cooking method that can help retain the nutritional value of food. Baked foods like sweet potatoes, squash, and carrots are rich in nutrients like vitamins A and C, which are beneficial for prostate health. Baking is also a good option for preparing lean protein sources like chicken or fish.

**Boiling:**

Boiling is a healthy cooking method that can help retain the nutritional value of food. When boiling vegetables like broccoli or kale, it is important to avoid overcooking them as this can reduce their nutritional value. To prevent overcooking, it is recommended to cook the vegetables for a short amount of time and then shock them in cold water to stop the cooking process.

In conclusion, choosing the right cooking methods can be beneficial for prostate health.

*Grilling, steaming, stir-frying, baking, and boiling* are all healthy cooking methods that can help retain the nutritional value of food. Incorporating a variety of cooked and raw vegetables, lean protein sources, and healthy fats into your diet can promote overall prostate health and reduce the risk of developing prostate cancer.

# CHAPTER 3

**Breakfast Recipes:**

Breakfast is considered the most important meal of the day, and it is important to start your day with a healthy, balanced meal. Here are some breakfast recipes that are both delicious and nutritious:

**Overnight oats:**

Overnight oats are a simple and easy breakfast option that can be prepared the night before. To make overnight oats, simply mix rolled oats with milk (or a non-dairy alternative), yogurt, and your favorite toppings like fruit, nuts, and honey. Let the mixture sit in the fridge overnight, and in the morning, you will have a delicious and filling breakfast ready to go.

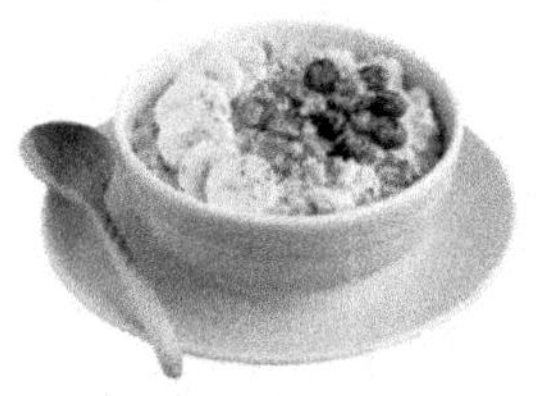

**Avocado toast:**

Avocado toast is a popular breakfast dish that is both delicious and nutritious. To make avocado toast, toast a slice of whole-grain bread and top it with mashed avocado, salt, and pepper. You can also add additional toppings like a fried egg or sliced tomatoes for extra flavor and nutrition.

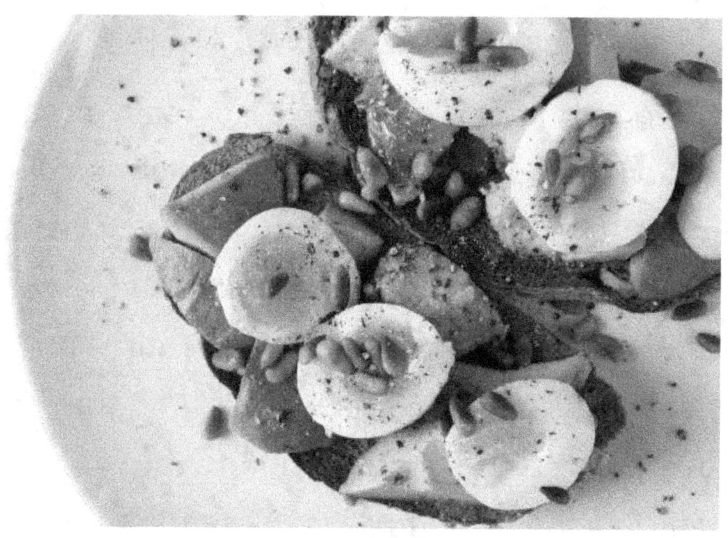

**Greek yogurt parfait:**

Greek yogurt parfaits are a great breakfast option for those who are on the go. Simply layer Greek yogurt with your favorite fruits and nuts in a jar or container, and you will have a delicious and healthy breakfast that you can take with you anywhere.

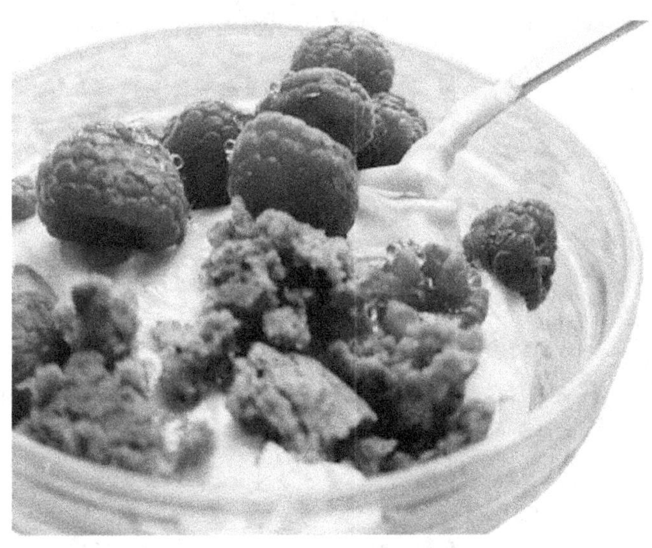

**Breakfast burrito:**

Breakfast burritos are a hearty and filling breakfast option that is perfect for those who need a more substantial meal in the morning. To make a breakfast burrito, scramble eggs with your favorite veggies like bell peppers, onions, and spinach. Add some shredded cheese and wrap the mixture in a whole-grain tortilla for a tasty and satisfying breakfast.

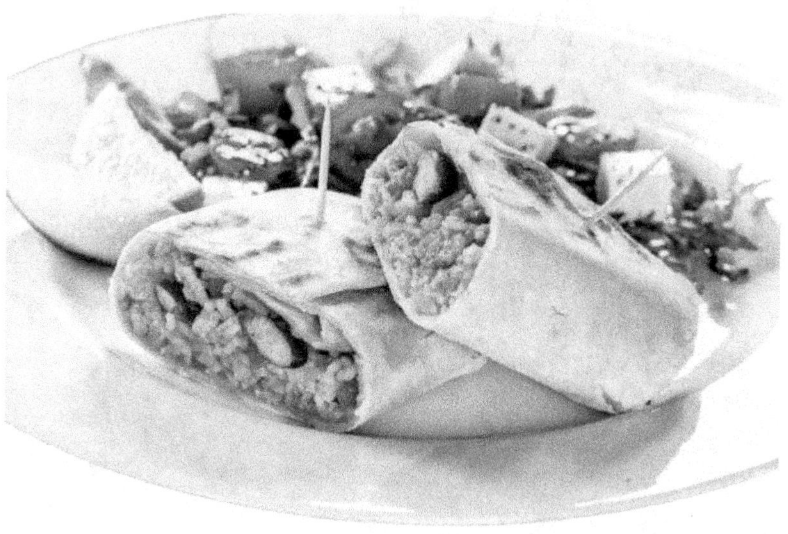

**Smoothie bowl:**

Smoothie bowls are a fun and colourful breakfast option that is perfect for those who love smoothies. To make a smoothie bowl, blend frozen fruits like berries or bananas with milk (or a non-dairy alternative) and your favourite protein powder. Pour the mixture into a bowl and top it with your favourite toppings like granola, chia seeds, and fresh fruit.

Breakfast is an important meal that should not be skipped. These breakfast recipes are easy to prepare, delicious, and packed with nutrients that can help fuel your day. By starting your day with a healthy and balanced breakfast, you can improve your overall health and wellbeing.

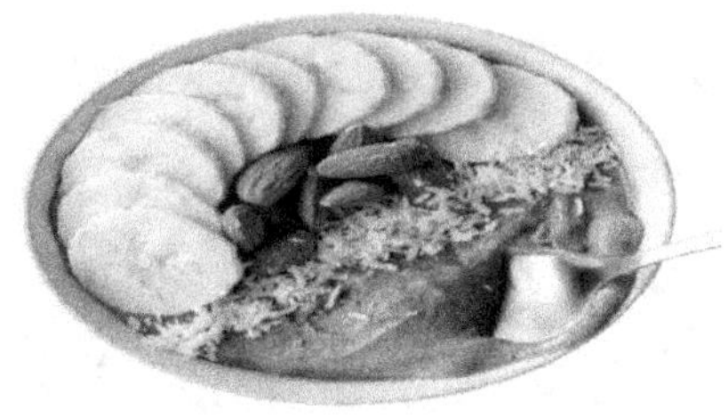

# CHAPTER 4

**Appetizers and Snacks**

Prostate health is an important concern for men, particularly as they age. The prostate gland is a walnut-sized gland located just below the bladder, and it plays a crucial role in the male reproductive system. As men age, their risk of developing prostate problems, such as prostate cancer, increases. However, making dietary changes and incorporating certain foods into your diet can help promote prostate health. In this article, we will focus on appetizers and snacks that can support prostate health.

**Nuts:** Nuts are an excellent source of healthy fats, fiber, and protein, making them a great snack option for prostate health. Walnuts, in particular, contain high levels of omega-3 fatty acids, which have been shown to reduce inflammation and lower the risk of prostate cancer.

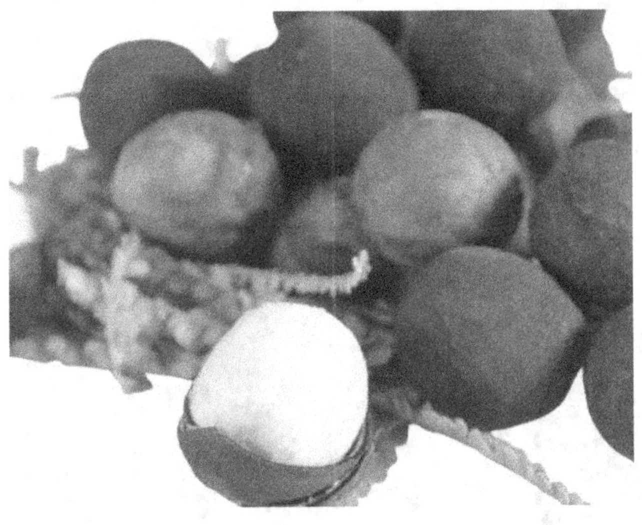

Seeds: Like nuts, seeds are also a great source of healthy fats, fiber, and protein. Pumpkin seeds, in particular, are high in zinc, which is important for prostate health. Studies have shown that a diet high in zinc may reduce the risk of developing prostate cancer.

**Tomatoes:** Tomatoes are high in lycopene, a powerful antioxidant that has been shown to reduce the risk of prostate cancer. Eating cooked tomatoes, such as in a tomato sauce, can actually increase the amount of lycopene your body absorbs.

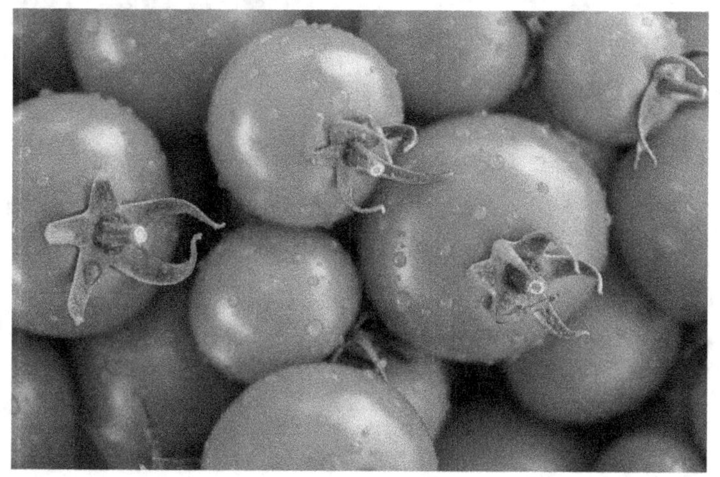

**Berries:** Berries are high in antioxidants, which can help protect the body against oxidative stress and inflammation. Blueberries, in particular, have been shown to have anti-cancer properties and may help reduce the risk of prostate cancer.

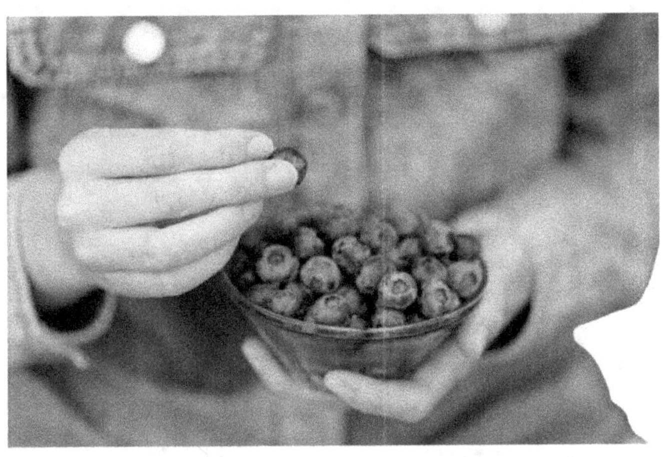

**Avocado:** Avocado is an excellent source of healthy fats, fiber, and potassium. It also contains beta-sitosterol, a compound that has been shown to improve urinary symptoms in men with an enlarged prostate.

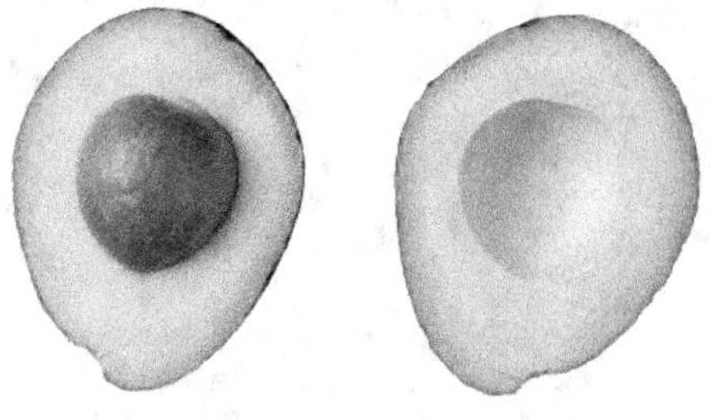

**Edamame**: Edamame, or soybeans, are a great source of protein, fiber, and several vitamins and minerals. Soybeans contain isoflavones, which are compounds that may help reduce the risk of prostate cancer.

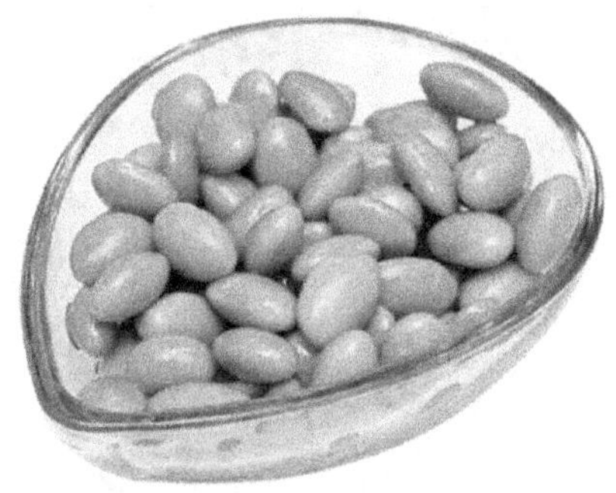

**Hummus**: Hummus is a great source of protein, fiber, and healthy fats. It's also high in zinc and vitamin B6, both of which are important for prostate health.

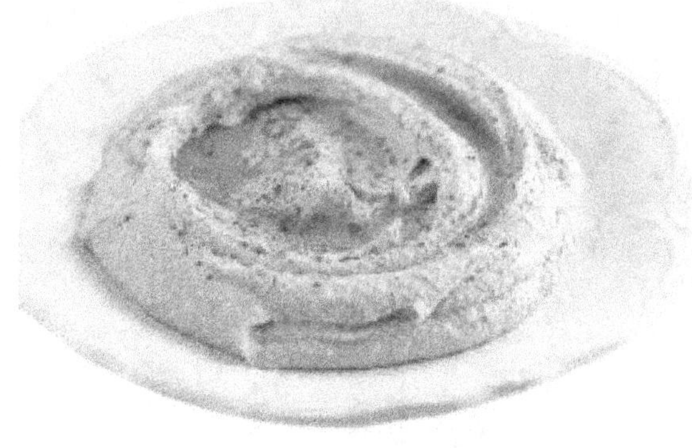

**Greek yogurt**: Greek yogurt is high in protein and calcium, which are both important for bone health. It also contains probiotics, which may help improve gut health and reduce inflammation in the body.

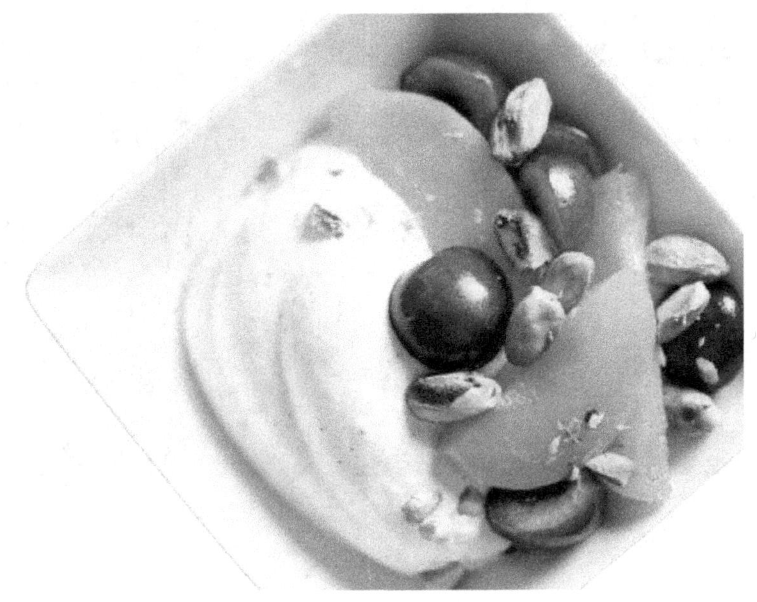

**Dark chocolate:** Dark chocolate is high in antioxidants and may help reduce inflammation in the body. Studies have also shown that consuming dark chocolate may help reduce the risk of prostate cancer.

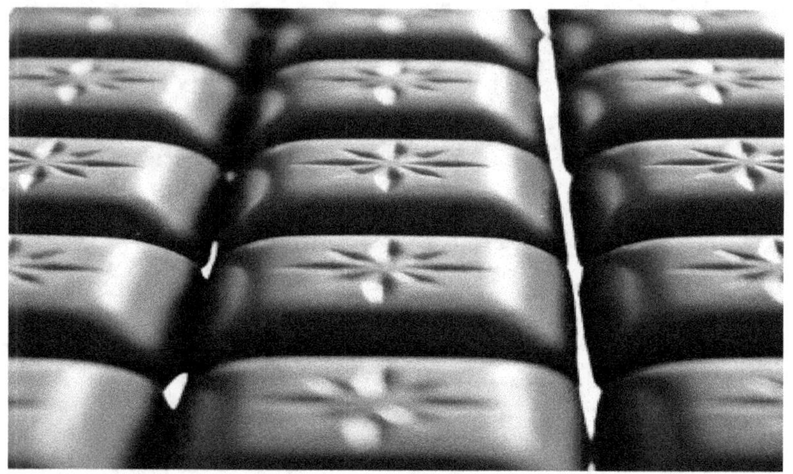

**Green tea:** Green tea is high in antioxidants and has been shown to have anti-cancer properties. Studies have also shown that drinking green tea may help reduce the risk of prostate cancer.

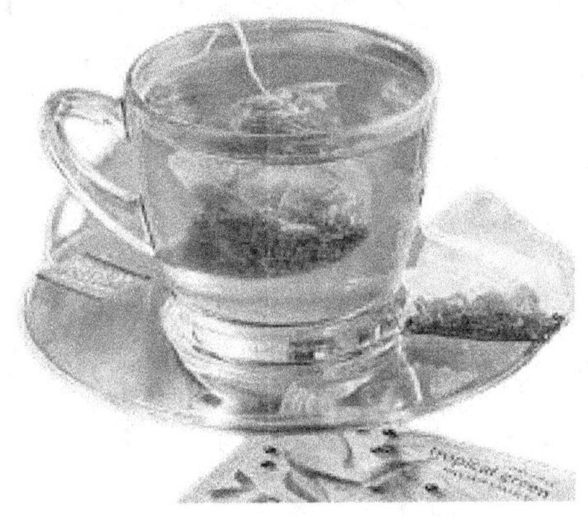

**Spicy Roasted Nuts**: Spicy Roasted Nuts" make for a delightful and prostate-friendly appetizer or snack, combining both flavor and nutritional benefits. Nuts, such as *almonds, walnuts, and pecans*, are excellent sources of healthy fats, essential for prostate health. The inclusion of spices like *cayenne pepper or chili powder* not only adds a zesty kick but may also contribute anti-inflammatory properties.

To prepare Spicy Roasted Nuts, coat a mix of your preferred nuts with a light drizzle of olive oil, ensuring an even coating. Sprinkle a blend of spices, including cayenne pepper, paprika, garlic powder, and a pinch of sea salt for added flavor. Spread the seasoned nuts on a baking sheet in a single layer and roast them in the oven until they achieve a golden brown hue and emit a fragrant aroma. Allow the nuts to cool before serving.

This appetizer not only satisfies your taste buds with its crunchy texture and bold flavors but also provides a healthy dose of nutrients beneficial for prostate health. Remember to practice moderation when enjoying these Spicy Roasted Nuts, as nuts are energy-dense, and a balanced approach ensures optimal health benefits.

**Beet Hummus**: star ingredient, not only lend a beautiful magenta hue but also pack a nutritional punch. Beets contain antioxidants, fiber, and essential vitamins, contributing to overall prostate health.

To prepare Beet Hummus, start by roasting or boiling fresh beets until tender. Once cooled, peel and chop the beets, and then combine them with *chickpeas, tahini, garlic, lemon juice, and olive oil* in a food processor. Blend until smooth, adjusting the consistency with water if needed. Season with salt and pepper to taste.

This prostate-conscious appetizer not only offers a unique flavor profile but also introduces additional health benefits. Beets have been associated with anti-inflammatory and antioxidant properties, potentially contributing to prostate health. Serve Beet Hummus with whole-grain crackers or vegetable sticks for a delicious and nutritious snack that supports your overall well-being.

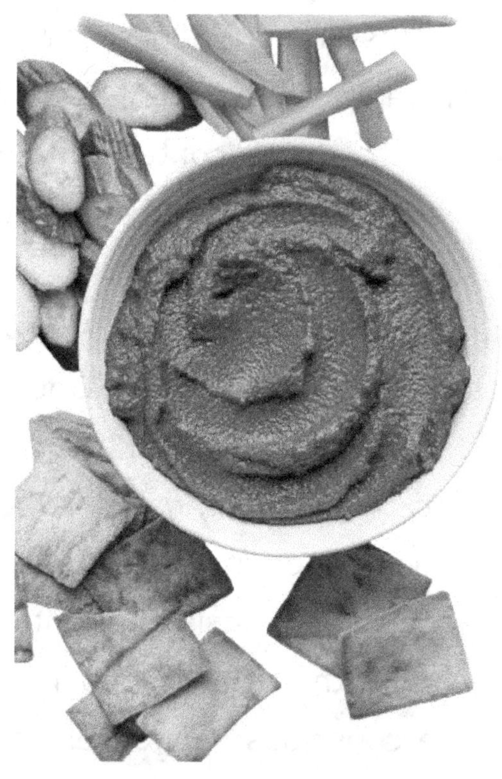

**Grilled Zucchini Rolls**: To prepare Grilled Zucchini Rolls, start by slicing zucchini lengthwise into thin strips. Lightly brush the zucchini with olive oil and season with salt and pepper. Grill the zucchini strips until they are tender and have distinct grill marks. For the stuffing, mix a combination of ingredients like *herbed cream cheese, sundried tomatoes, and fresh basil*. Spread the filling onto each grilled zucchini strip, then roll them up into bite-sized rolls.

These zesty and visually appealing rolls not only provide a burst of flavor but also contribute to prostate health with the inclusion of zucchini, which contains essential nutrients and antioxidants. Serve Grilled Zucchini Rolls as an appetizer or snack, showcasing a delicious way to incorporate prostate-friendly ingredients into your culinary repertoire.

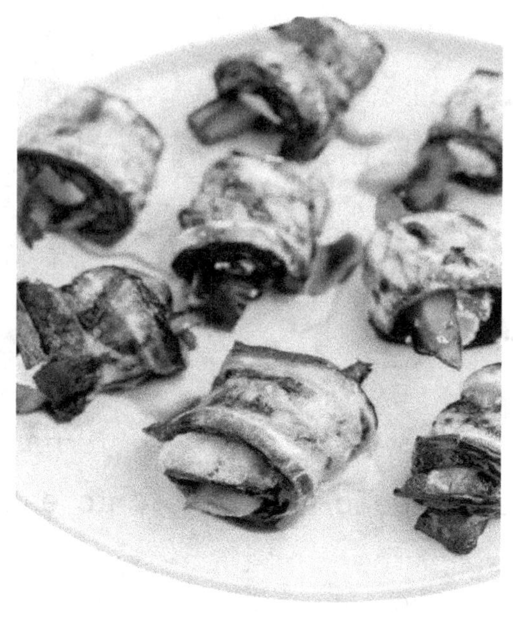

In conclusion, incorporating these appetizers and snacks into your diet can help support prostate health. However, it's important to remember that a healthy diet alone cannot prevent or treat prostate problems. It's also important to maintain a healthy lifestyle by exercising regularly, maintaining a healthy weight, and getting regular check-ups with your doctor.

# CHAPTER 5

**Salads and Dressings:**

Salads and dressings are a popular and healthy option for those looking to maintain a nutritious diet. A salad typically consists of a mixture of fresh vegetables, fruits, nuts, and seeds, while dressings are used to add flavor and moisture to the salad. In this comprehensive note, we will discuss salads and dressings, their benefits, and some tips for making them.

**Benefits of Salads:**

**Nutrient-rich:** Salads are packed with vitamins, minerals, and antioxidants that are essential for maintaining good health.

**Low in Calories**: Salads are typically low in calories and high in fiber, making them a great option for weight loss and management.

Easy to prepare: Salads are quick and easy to prepare, and can be made with a variety of fresh ingredients.

**Types of Salads:**

**Green salads**: These are made primarily from leafy greens such as lettuce, kale, and spinach.

**Vegetable salads:** These salads are made from a variety of vegetables such as tomatoes, cucumbers, carrots, and peppers.

**Fruit salads:** These salads are made from a variety of fruits such as strawberries, blueberries, oranges, and apples.

**Grain salads**: These salads are made from grains such as quinoa, couscous, or bulgur and often include vegetables and herbs.

**Benefits of Dressings:**

Adds flavor: Dressings add flavor to salads and can be used to enhance the natural flavors of the ingredients.

Provides moisture: Dressings provide moisture to salads, making them easier to eat and more enjoyable.

Nutritious: Many dressings are made with healthy fats and ingredients such as olive oil, vinegar, and herbs, which provide health benefits.

**Types of Dressings:**

**Vinaigrette:** Made with olive oil, vinegar, and seasonings, this dressing is light and tangy.

**Ranch:** Made with buttermilk, mayonnaise, and seasonings, this dressing is creamy and flavorful.

**Caesar:** Made with olive oil, garlic, lemon juice, and anchovies, this dressing is tangy and savory.

**Balsamic**: Made with balsamic vinegar, olive oil, and seasonings, this dressing is sweet and tangy.

**Tips for making Salads and Dressings:**
Choose fresh ingredients: Use fresh, high-quality ingredients for the best flavor and nutrition.

Mix and match: Mix and match different types of vegetables, fruits, nuts, and seeds to create a variety of salads.

Be creative with dressings: Experiment with different types of dressings to find your favorite flavors.

**Use healthy fats**: Use healthy fats such as olive oil, avocado, or nuts in dressings to provide health benefits.

**Balance flavors**: Be sure to balance sweet, salty, and sour flavors in both salads and dressings to create a well-rounded flavor profile.

In conclusion, salads and dressings are a delicious and healthy option for those looking to maintain a nutritious diet. With a wide variety of ingredients and flavors to choose from, they offer endless possibilities for creating tasty and satisfying meals.

Rainbow Salad with Ginger Dressing

Grilled Chicken Salad

Caesar Salad with Homemade Dressing

# CHAPTER 6

**Soups and Stews:**

Soups and stews are a healthy and delicious way to incorporate a variety of ingredients into your diet, including those that may be beneficial for prostate health. The prostate gland is a small organ located near the bladder and is an important part of the male reproductive system. As men age, the prostate gland can become enlarged and lead to a condition known as benign prostatic hyperplasia (BPH) or even prostate cancer.

Incorporating certain foods into your diet can potentially reduce your risk of developing these conditions. Here are some ingredients commonly found in soups and stews that may be beneficial for prostate health:

**Tomatoes:** Tomatoes contain lycopene, a powerful antioxidant that has been linked to a reduced risk of prostate cancer. Cooking tomatoes actually increases the bioavailability of lycopene, making them an excellent addition to soups and stews.

**Cruciferous vegetables:** Vegetables like broccoli, cauliflower, and kale are rich in compounds called glucosinolates, which can help the body detoxify and potentially reduce the risk of prostate cancer.

**Legumes:** Beans and lentils are rich in fiber, which can help regulate bowel movements and reduce the risk of constipation, a risk factor for prostate problems. They also contain plant-based proteins, which are important for overall health.

**Turmeric:** Turmeric contains curcumin, a compound with anti-inflammatory properties that has been shown to reduce the risk of prostate cancer and BPH.

**Garlic and onions:** These vegetables contain sulfur compounds that can potentially reduce inflammation in the body and reduce the risk of prostate cancer.

When it comes to preparing soups and stews for prostate health, it's important to use healthy cooking methods like boiling or simmering, which can help retain the nutrients in the ingredients. Avoid using excessive salt, as too much sodium can increase blood pressure and potentially exacerbate prostate problems.

In summary, incorporating a variety of nutrient-rich ingredients into soups and stews can be an excellent way to support prostate health. By including ingredients like tomatoes, cruciferous vegetables, legumes, turmeric, garlic, and onions, you can potentially reduce your risk of developing prostate problems and improve your overall health and wellbeing.

<h1 style="text-align:center">CHAPTER 7</h1>

**Seafood:**

Seafood is a rich source of various nutrients, including omega-3 fatty acids, which have been linked to several health benefits, including prostate health. The prostate gland is an important part of the male reproductive system, and as men age, they are at an increased risk of developing prostate problems, such as benign prostatic hyperplasia (BPH) or prostate cancer. Here are some ways in which seafood can potentially benefit prostate health:

**Omega-3 fatty acids:** Fatty fish such as salmon, mackerel, and sardines are rich in omega-3 fatty acids, which have anti-inflammatory properties and can potentially reduce the risk of prostate cancer and BPH. Some studies have found that men who consume higher amounts of omega-3 fatty acids have a lower risk of developing prostate cancer.

**Selenium:** Seafood is a good source of selenium, an essential mineral that has been linked to a reduced risk of prostate cancer. Selenium can also help reduce inflammation in the body, which is a risk factor for prostate problems.

**Vitamin D:** Fatty fish is also a good source of vitamin D, which has been linked to a reduced risk of prostate cancer. Vitamin D can also help maintain bone health and boost the immune system.

**Zinc:** Some types of seafood, such as oysters, are a rich source of zinc, which is important for prostate health. Zinc has been shown to help reduce the size of an enlarged prostate gland and improve urinary symptoms associated with BPH.

When it comes to preparing seafood for prostate health, it's important to choose healthy cooking methods, such as baking, grilling, or steaming, instead of frying. Avoid consuming high amounts of mercury-containing seafood, such as shark, swordfish, and king mackerel, which can potentially harm prostate health.

In summary, seafood is a rich source of nutrients that can potentially benefit prostate health. Omega-3 fatty acids, selenium, vitamin D, and zinc are all important nutrients that have been linked to a reduced risk of prostate problems. By incorporating seafood into a balanced diet and using healthy cooking methods, men can potentially reduce their risk of developing prostate problems and improve their overall health and wellbeing.

# CHAPTER 8

## Poultry

Poultry, such as chicken and turkey, can be a healthy and nutritious addition to a balanced diet. When it comes to prostate health, there are a few key benefits to incorporating poultry into your meals.

**High in Protein**: Poultry is an excellent source of high-quality protein, which is essential for maintaining muscle mass and overall health. Protein also plays a role in maintaining healthy hormone levels, which can help support prostate health.

**Low in Saturated Fat**: Compared to red meat, poultry is generally lower in saturated fat. Diets high in saturated fat have been linked to an increased risk of prostate cancer, so choosing leaner protein sources like poultry can be a healthier option.

**Rich in Vitamins and Minerals**: Poultry is a good source of a variety of vitamins and minerals, including B vitamins, selenium, and zinc. These nutrients can support overall health and potentially benefit prostate health as well.

Here are some examples of healthy and delicious ways to incorporate poultry into your diet:

**Grilled Chicken with Vegetables**: Marinate chicken breasts in a mixture of olive oil, lemon juice, garlic, and herbs, then grill them alongside your favorite vegetables for a healthy and flavorful meal.

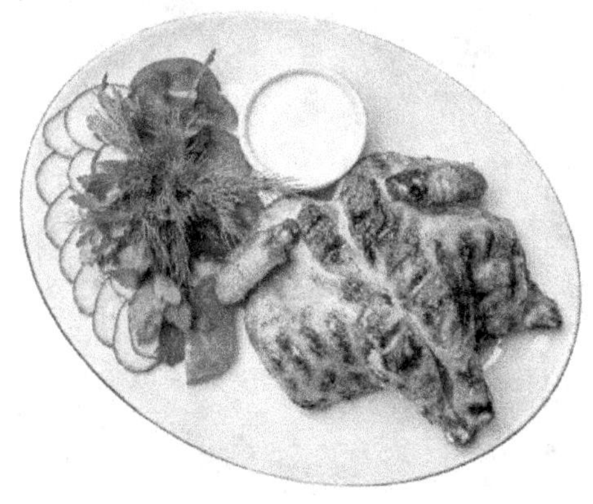

**Turkey Chili**: Use ground turkey in place of beef for a leaner and healthier version of classic chili. Add plenty of vegetables like tomatoes, onions, and peppers for added nutrition.

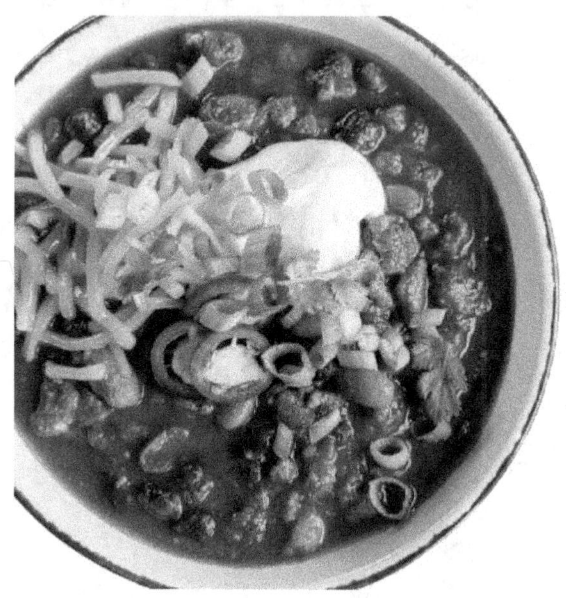

**Chicken Stir-Fry:** Stir-fry chicken breast with a variety of vegetables like broccoli, bell peppers, and mushrooms. Serve over quinoa or brown rice for a satisfying and wholesome dinner.

When purchasing poultry, look for lean cuts and choose organic or free-range options when possible. It's also important to cook poultry to a safe internal temperature to avoid foodborne illness. By incorporating poultry into your diet in a healthy and balanced way, you can potentially support prostate health while enjoying delicious and nutritious meals.

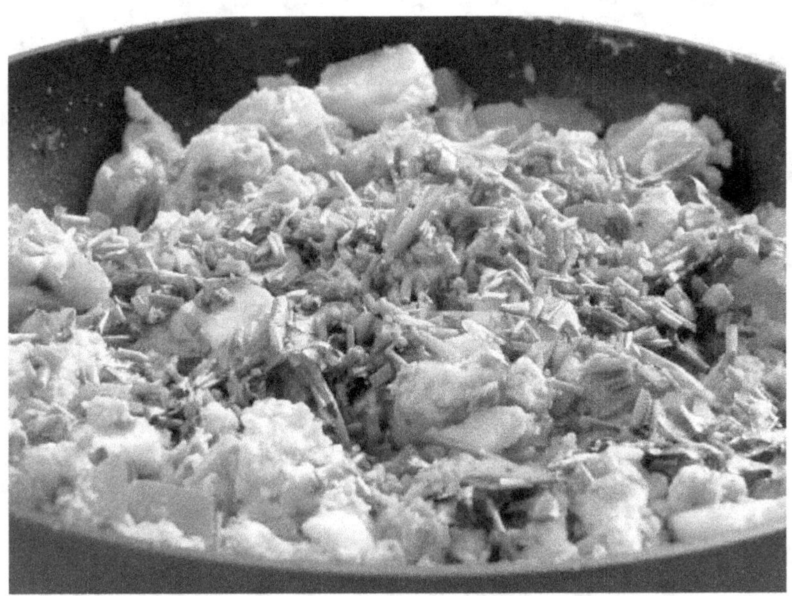

# CHAPTER 9

**Meat:**

Meat is a valuable source of protein and other essential nutrients, but it has been associated with various health concerns, including prostate cancer. The second most prevalent form of cancer in men worldwide and the fifth most frequent cause of cancer death is prostate cancer. There is evidence suggesting that a high intake of meat, especially red and processed meat, may increase the risk of developing prostate cancer. In this context, it is important to understand the relationship between meat consumption and prostate health.

Red meat, such as *beef, pork, and lamb*, contains a high amount of saturated fat and cholesterol, which may increase the risk of developing prostate cancer. A study published in the American Journal of Epidemiology reported that men who consumed high amounts of red meat had a 12% higher risk of developing prostate cancer compared to men who consumed less red meat. Similarly, a study published in the Journal of the National Cancer Institute found that men who consumed high amounts of processed meat had a 50% higher risk of developing prostate cancer compared to men who consumed less processed meat.

On the other hand, poultry, such as chicken and turkey, contains less saturated fat and cholesterol than red meat and may have a lower association with prostate cancer. In fact, a study published in the Journal of the American Medical Association found that men who consumed poultry had a lower risk of developing prostate cancer compared to men who consumed red meat.

Fish, especially fatty fish such as salmon and tuna, are excellent sources of omega-3 fatty acids, which have anti-inflammatory properties and may reduce the risk of developing prostate cancer. A study published in the International Journal of Cancer found that men who consumed high amounts of fish had a 44% lower risk of developing prostate cancer compared to men who consumed low amounts of fish.

Additionally, here are some examples of meat-based dishes that can be included in a healthy diet that supports prostate health:

**Beef and Vegetable Stir-Fry**: This dish is a great way to incorporate lean beef and a variety of vegetables into your diet. Start by marinating beef strips in a mixture of soy sauce, rice vinegar, and garlic. Then, stir-fry the beef in a wok or skillet with vegetables such as broccoli, bell peppers, and onions. Assemble a nutritious and satisfying meal by serving over brown rice.

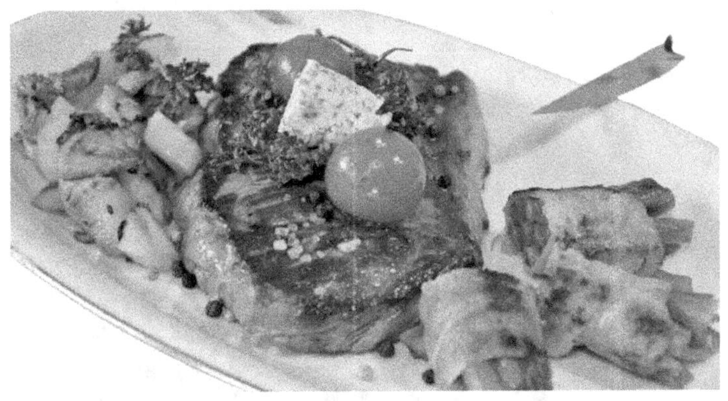

**Lamb Chops with Mint Sauce:** Lamb is a good source of protein and iron, and when paired with a refreshing mint sauce, it can be a delicious and healthy meal option. Simply season lamb chops with salt and pepper, and grill or pan-sear until cooked to your desired doneness. For the mint sauce, mix together chopped fresh mint, lemon juice, garlic, and olive oil. Serve the lamb chops with the mint sauce and a side of roasted vegetables.

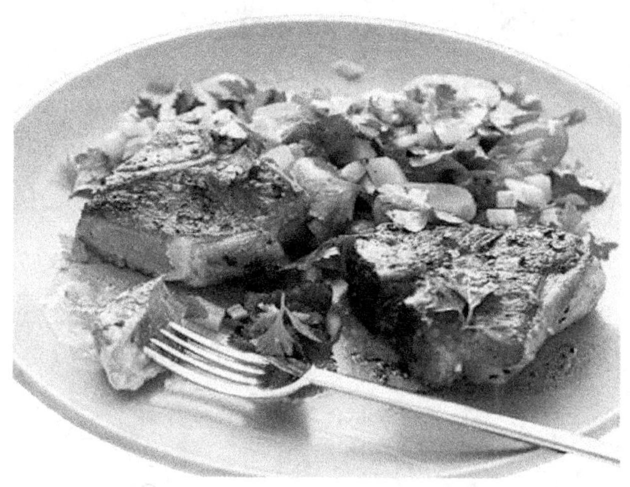

**Grilled Steak with Chimichurri Sauce**: Grilling is a healthy cooking method that helps to retain the nutrients and flavor of meat. For this recipe, marinate a steak in a mixture of olive oil, garlic, and lime juice. Then, grill the meat until it is cooked as you prefer. For the chimichurri sauce, blend together fresh parsley, garlic, red wine vinegar, and olive oil. Serve the grilled steak with the chimichurri sauce and a side of grilled vegetables.

It is important to note that while these dishes contain meat, they also incorporate a variety of vegetables and healthy fats, which are important components of a balanced and healthy diet. Incorporating a variety of meats, as well as fish and poultry, into your diet in moderation, and pairing them with vegetables and healthy fats, can help support prostate health and overall well-being.

In conclusion, while meat is an important source of protein and nutrients, especially for people who follow a low-carbohydrate diet, it is important to consume it in moderation and choose lean sources of meat such as poultry and fish. A diet rich in fruits, vegetables, whole grains, and healthy fats such as olive oil and nuts has been associated with a lower risk of developing prostate cancer. It is also recommended to limit the consumption of red and processed meat to reduce the risk of prostate cancer and other health concerns.

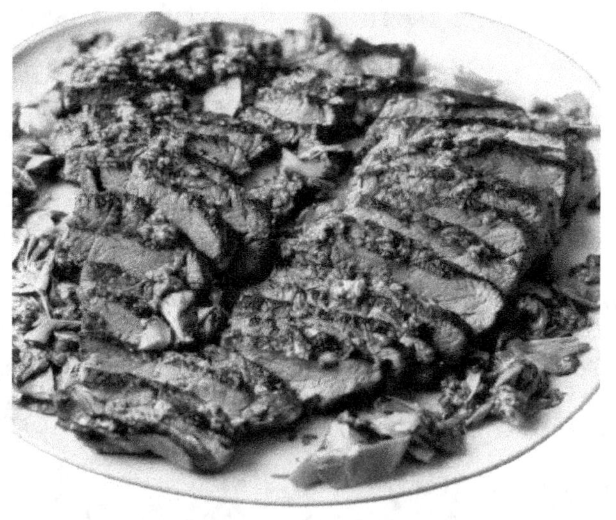

# CHAPTER 10

**Vegetarian and Vegan:**

A vegetarian or vegan diet can provide a wide range of health benefits, including a reduced risk of chronic diseases such as heart disease, diabetes, and some types of cancer. However, it is important to consider the potential impact of a vegetarian or vegan diet on prostate health.

Research has suggested that vegetarian and vegan diets may have a protective effect on prostate health. For example, a study published in the American Journal of Clinical Nutrition found that men who followed a vegan or vegetarian diet had a lower risk of developing prostate cancer compared to men who consumed meat. Another study published in the journal Urology found that men who followed a vegan diet had a lower risk of developing prostate cancer compared to men who consumed a Western-style diet high in meat and fat.

Vegetarian and vegan diets are typically rich in fruits, vegetables, whole grains, legumes, and nuts, which provide a variety of nutrients and antioxidants that can support prostate health. For example, lycopene, which is found in tomatoes and other red fruits and vegetables, has been associated with a lower risk of prostate cancer. Additionally, plant-based sources of protein, such as legumes, tofu, and tempeh, can provide the necessary protein intake without the potentially harmful effects of consuming too much animal protein.

However, it is important for vegetarians and vegans to ensure that they are getting sufficient amounts of certain nutrients that are typically found in animal products. For example, vitamin B12, which is necessary for nerve and red blood cell health, is primarily found in animal products. Vegetarians and vegans may need to supplement their diet with vitamin B12 or consume fortified foods to ensure adequate intake.

Here are some examples of vegetarian and vegan dishes that can be included in a healthy diet that supports prostate health:

**Chickpea and Sweet Potato Curry:** This dish is a delicious and hearty way to incorporate legumes and vegetables into your diet. Simply sauté onions, garlic, and ginger in a large pot, and then add diced sweet potatoes and chickpeas. Pour in coconut milk and vegetable broth, and let the curry simmer until the sweet potatoes are tender. Serve over brown rice or with naan bread for a satisfying meal.

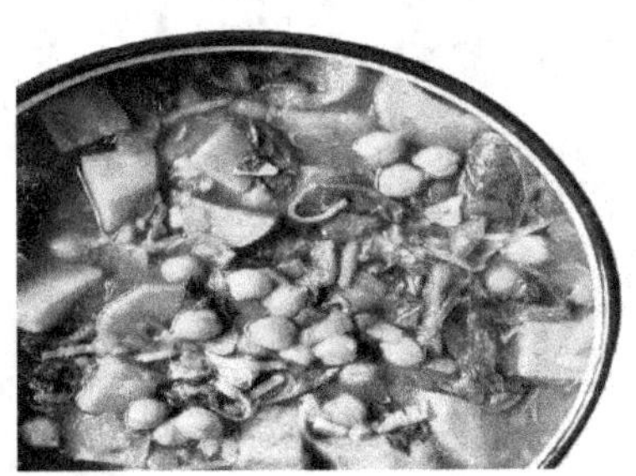

**Lentil Shepherd's Pie:** This dish is a healthy and flavorful take on the classic comfort food. Start by cooking lentils in a mixture of vegetable broth, diced onions, and garlic. Then, layer the lentil mixture with mashed sweet potatoes or cauliflower in a baking dish, and bake until the top is golden brown. This dish is rich in fiber and plant-based protein, making it a great addition to a prostate-healthy diet.

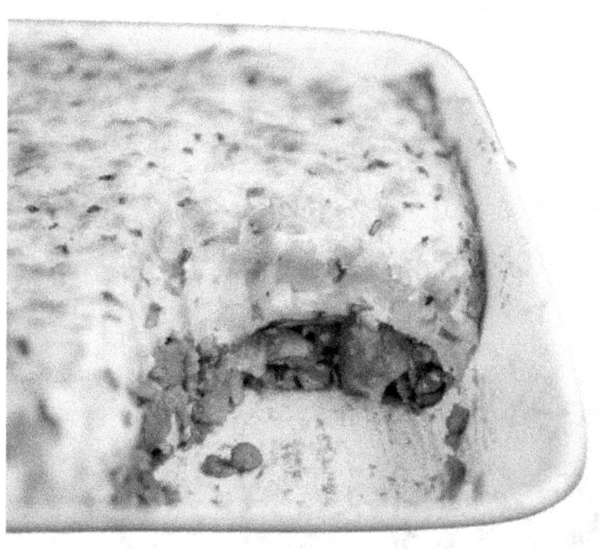

**Roasted Vegetable Pasta:** This dish is a simple and flavorful way to incorporate a variety of vegetables into your diet. Simply toss your favorite vegetables in olive oil and roast them in the oven until tender. Then, toss the vegetables with whole-grain pasta and a sauce made from blended roasted red peppers, garlic, and basil. This dish is rich in antioxidants and fiber, and can be customized to your taste preferences.

It is important to note that while these dishes are vegetarian or vegan, they still provide a variety of nutrients that are important for prostate health. Legumes and vegetables are excellent sources of fiber and antioxidants, which have been associated with a reduced risk of chronic diseases, including prostate cancer. By incorporating a variety of plant-based foods into your diet, you can support prostate health and overall well-being.

In conclusion, a well-planned vegetarian or vegan diet can provide a wide range of health benefits, including a reduced risk of prostate cancer. However, it is important to ensure that the diet includes a variety of nutrient-dense foods, including sources of protein and important micronutrients. Consulting with a registered dietitian can help ensure that a vegetarian or vegan diet is balanced and meets individual nutrient needs.

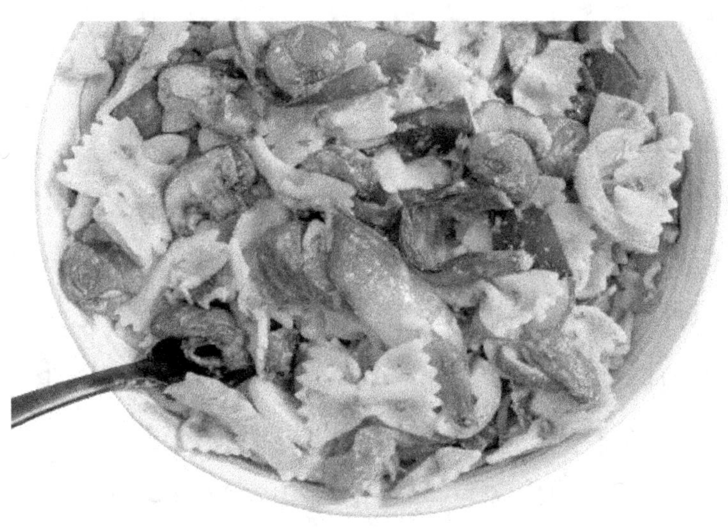

# CHAPTER 11

**Desserts**

Desserts can be a delicious and satisfying way to end a meal, but it is important to choose options that support prostate health. Here are some examples of desserts that can be enjoyed as part of a balanced and prostate-healthy diet:

**Fresh fruit:** Fresh fruit is a delicious and nutritious way to satisfy a sweet tooth. Fruits like berries, oranges, and pomegranates are particularly high in antioxidants, which can help protect against prostate cancer. Serve sliced fruit with a dollop of yogurt or a drizzle of honey for a simple and healthy dessert.

**Dark chocolate:** Dark chocolate is rich in antioxidants and flavonoids, which have been associated with a reduced risk of chronic diseases, including prostate cancer. Choose dark chocolate that contains at least 70% cocoa solids, and enjoy a small serving as a treat after a meal.

**Yogurt parfait**: Yogurt is a great source of protein and probiotics, which can support gut health and overall well-being. Layer Greek yogurt with fresh fruit, granola, and a drizzle of honey for a delicious and healthy dessert.

**Baked apples**: Baked apples are a delicious and comforting dessert that can be enjoyed warm or cold. Simply slice apples and bake in the oven with a sprinkle of cinnamon and a drizzle of honey until tender and golden brown. Serve with a dollop of Greek yogurt for a protein-rich dessert.

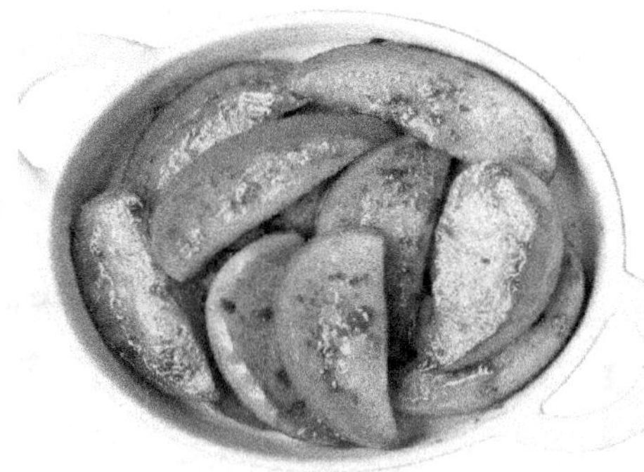

**Chia seed pudding:** Chia seeds are a great source of fiber and healthy fats, and can be used to make a delicious and healthy pudding. Simply mix chia seeds with coconut milk, vanilla extract, and a sweetener of your choice, and let the mixture sit in the fridge until thick and creamy. Serve with fresh fruit for a satisfying and nutritious dessert.

By choosing desserts that are rich in antioxidants, fiber, and healthy fats, you can support prostate health and overall well-being. Aim to incorporate a variety of colorful fruits, dark chocolate, yogurt, and healthy seeds into your desserts to ensure a balanced and prostate-healthy diet.

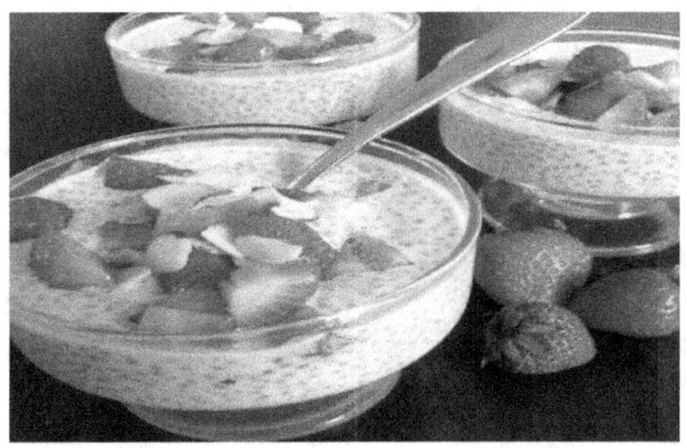

## Conclusion

In conclusion, prostate health is a critical aspect of men's overall well-being. As men age, the prostate gland undergoes changes that can lead to various health issues, such as prostate cancer, prostatitis, and benign prostatic hyperplasia (BPH). Therefore, it is essential to maintain good prostate health through a healthy lifestyle and regular medical check-ups.

Several lifestyle factors can promote good prostate health, including a balanced diet rich in *fruits, vegetables, and lean protein, regular exercise, maintaining a healthy weight, limiting alcohol consumption, and quitting smoking.* These healthy lifestyle choices can also reduce the risk of developing other chronic conditions such as cardiovascular disease and diabetes, which can also affect prostate health.

Regular medical check-ups, including a prostate-specific antigen (PSA) test and a digital rectal exam (DRE), can help detect prostate problems early when they are easier to treat. Men should discuss their prostate health with their healthcare provider and understand the risks and benefits of prostate cancer screening tests.

In summary, taking care of prostate health is crucial for men's overall well-being. A healthy lifestyle, including a balanced diet, regular exercise, and regular medical check-ups, can reduce the risk of prostate problems and other chronic conditions, helping men to live healthy and fulfilling lives.

**Tips for incorporating prostate-healthy foods into your diet:**

Incorporating prostate-healthy foods into your diet is an effective way to support good prostate health. Here are some tips for incorporating prostate-healthy foods into your diet:

**Start with small changes**: Making small changes to your diet can be easier to stick with than trying to overhaul your entire diet at once. Start by incorporating one prostate-healthy food into your diet each week, and gradually add more over time.

**Plan your meals**: Plan your meals ahead of time to ensure that you have prostate-healthy foods on hand. This can help you avoid reaching for less healthy options when you're hungry and pressed for time.

**Experiment with different recipes**: Try new recipes that incorporate prostate-healthy foods. This can help keep your meals interesting and prevent boredom with your diet.

Add prostate-healthy foods to your favorite recipes: Look for ways to add prostate-healthy foods to your favorite recipes. For example, add tomatoes to your favorite pasta sauce or top your salad with nuts.

**Snack on prostate-healthy foods**: Keep prostate-healthy snacks on hand, such as berries or nuts, to help you stay full and satisfied between meals.

**Opt for healthy cooking methods**: Use healthy cooking methods such as *grilling, broiling, and baking* to help preserve the nutritional value of prostate-healthy foods.

**Be mindful of portion sizes:** While prostate-healthy foods are beneficial, it's important to be mindful of portion sizes. Eating too much of any food can lead to weight gain and other health problems.

In summary, incorporating prostate-healthy foods into your diet is a simple yet effective way to support good prostate health. By starting with small changes, planning your meals, experimenting with different recipes, adding prostate-healthy foods to your favorite recipes, snacking on prostate-healthy foods, opting for healthy cooking methods, and being mindful of portion sizes, you can make healthy eating a part of your lifestyle and support good prostate health.

**Additional resources for prostate health**

Here are some additional resources for prostate health:

**American Cancer Society**: The American Cancer Society provides information on prostate cancer, including risk factors, early detection, and treatment options. Their website also includes resources for patients and caregivers.

**Prostate Cancer Foundation**: The Prostate Cancer Foundation is dedicated to funding research to improve the prevention, detection, and treatment of prostate cancer. Their website provides information on prostate cancer and resources for patients and caregivers.

**Men's Health Network:** The Men's Health Network is a non-profit organization that focuses on promoting men's health and wellness. Their website includes information on prostate health and resources for men and their families.

National Institute of Diabetes and Digestive and Kidney Diseases (NIDDK): The NIDDK provides information on benign prostatic hyperplasia (BPH), including symptoms, diagnosis, and treatment options.

**Centres for Disease Control and Prevention (CDC):** The CDC provides information on prostate health, including risk factors, early detection, and screening guidelines.

**Prostate Cancer UK**: Prostate Cancer UK is a UK-based charity that provides information on prostate cancer and supports men and their families affected by the disease. Their website includes resources for patients and caregivers.

**Urology Care Foundation**: The Urology Care Foundation is a non-profit organization that provides information on urologic diseases, including prostate cancer, BPH, and prostatitis. Their website includes resources for patients and caregivers.

These resources can provide valuable information on prostate health and help individuals make informed decisions about their health. It's important to always consult with a healthcare provider for personalized advice and recommendations regarding prostate health.

www.ingramcontent.com/pod-product-compliance
Lightning Source LLC
Chambersburg PA
CBHW070833260726
48660CB00005B/2034